KILLER CALVES

THE ESSENTIAL GUIDE TO CALF GROWTH AND DEVELOPMENT

RHYS LARSON

BEASTLY BODY

CONTENTS

PREFACE

A few words of caution and encouragement.

This book is about helping you reach your potential, and getting your calves to grow.

Although pushing your limits helps you—and your calves—grow and improve, you should exercise thoughtfully and with common sense.

As you work to build your calves, don't take unnecessary risks or push yourself too hard, especially not to the point of injury.

Please consult a physician before embarking on any exercise program, especially if you have any questions or concerns about your body, your health, or your exercise limitations, and please do not do these exercises except under medical guidance if you usually don't specifically exercise your calves at all.

I want you **healthy** and exercising, rather than injured and exercising or not exercising at all!

It's the only way for those stubborn calves to actually benefit and grow.

—Rhys Larson

KILLER CALVES

Not everyone is born with the calves of their dreams. Whether you want calves that are well-formed, defined, supple, huge, or ripped, *Killer Calves* can help make your dreams a reality.

For those who want to banish their chicken legs to the distant past, *Killer Calves* will help turn your shrimpy calves into raging bulls.

If you want to be fit, bring variety to your exercise routines, add some lower leg development, or maintain what you have already worked so hard to attain, *Killer Calves* is for you too.

Killer Calves offers a wide range of tools, exercises, insights, and ideas to help shape your legs, particularly your calves.

So, if you're a hard gainer who has tried everything—or think you have—to build your calves, *Killer Calves* will give you numerous new ways to push your limits and help your muscles grow. If you're looking to sculpt and tone your lower legs, *Killer Calves* will provide you with a host of options to achieve the look you're after. Or, if you're already jacked and looking to add a bit of variety and new options to your leg routine, *Killer Calves* will give you novel ideas and programs to torture yourself at home and the gym.

Whether you're a fitness beginner looking for help, a seasoned bodybuilder or fitness professional looking for that little edge, someone who wants to get in shape, or an exercise enthusiast looking for a new approach, *Killer Calves* will help you improve your legs.

Everyone deserves a great pair of legs.

Everyone deserves a pair of killer calves!

HOW THIS BOOK WORKS

Killer Calves has been devised around the idea of giving you all the necessary knowledge and tools to get your calves to grow and develop the way you'd like them to.

To do this, *Killer Calves* is broken into sections that will give you numerous tips and exercise routines to try out. The options include basic exercises you may already know to off-the-wall ideas you've never heard of, much less tried.

These routines can be performed on their own or combined with other exercise programs. Added into your leg days, the exercises detailed here in *Killer Calves* will deliver so much more of an impact and intensity than just your standard calf circuit.

More than just your regular exercises and routines, *Killer Calves* will also provide you with differing techniques and variations for each exercise. These aim toward maximizing growth and training effectiveness, simultaneously delivering useful background information on basic anatomy and how the calves function, helping you understand how to best achieve the calf development you're seeking.

Finally—and this is a major inspiration for writing *Killer Calves*—by bringing all these ideas and approaches together in one place, I hope it will inspire you to experiment, explore, and learn which approaches work best for you. By learning techniques you'll love and value, I hope you will share how to get killer calves with anyone who's needing a boost to their leg game or struggling to meet their fitness goals.

Remember, the end goal of the calf development odyssey is yours to choose—whether it's colossal calves or simply sleek, defined, well-proportioned legs. Whatever outcome you decide, *Killer Calves* is here to make those goals possible.

CALFCENTRIC DEDICATION

Don't let anyone tell you that training your calves is easy. More than most other body parts, getting your calves to grow can be demanding, frustrating, and taxing. For some, the quest for calf development can even become all-consuming.

And, like almost anything worthwhile, getting the calves of your dreams requires dedication and hard work.

Lots of it.

This process is also not simple or quick, so if you came here hoping to land on a quick fix for your chicken legs, you're going to be disappointed. But don't give up!

Killer Calves will give you tools to help your calves grow through numerous ways to attack your weakest link and stimulate improvement.

But as with anything else worthwhile, you have to be dedicated to bring about change. You have to be committed and put forth the necessary effort.

Simply reading and understanding a workout, or going through the motions as you exercise will not get you where you want to be. Just signing up to the gym with a view to putting these exercises through their paces won't do a thing for you if you never attend and put yourself through the recommended exercises—and often.

Realize in the first place that your calves are used and worked every day, and so are resilient and resistant to change. To overcome this challenge, you have to be just as dedicated and determined as your calves are stubborn and reluctant. Essentially, you're going head to head with your stubborn calves and not taking no for an answer!

You have to counter their resistance to growth, and believe me, they will seem to throw out plenty of excuses along the way. But again, no amount of knowledge or range of exercises will do anything for you *if you don't make them count.*

And you are the only one who can do that for yourself.

Killer Calves will get you started on your way to the legs of your dreams, *but you are the one who has to get there…* one calf raise at a time.

Just in case you chose not to read the above, let's say again:

You are the one who has to get there. Nobody else can do it for you.

Train diligently, persevere, and embody your end goals with every repetition. Push yourself to reach your dreams because no one else will do it for you.

And then you, too, will have killer calves.

CALF PRIORITIZATION

Not only does training your calves require "calfcentric" focus and attention, but also, developing your calves requires prioritization. If you want to turn a weakness into a strength, you have to devote yourself to change, working creatively and strategically toward turning your liability into an asset, and putting forth the effort and dedication to see your goals through.

If calves are your weakness, you have to make them a priority.

It's that simple.

Think of the problem of helping your calves grow and develop in terms of common workout programs and goals... normal fitness frameworks and paradigms. People go to the gym all the time, primarily for their chest days, back days, and arm days.

But how often do people go to the gym for calf days?

Even on leg days, calves are often an afterthought if they're worked at all, and far too often neglected.

When your gym buddies are bragging about their latest workout or new routine, chances are they are not talking about their calves or everything they did on calf day. There are so many articles in books, magazines, and online, focusing on every single other body part... except calf day.

Sure, there are articles on calf exercises and programs, but the calves are generally treated as a secondary muscle group to be incorporated into a leg workout or as an afterthought.

With *Killer Calves*, I'm here to change that.

Together, we're going to make calves a priority.

We're going to make every day calf day!

CALF EXERCISE OVERVIEW

Before diving into the exercises, programs, and concepts presented in *Killer Calves*, here's a brief overview of the exercise types you'll use to add life, definition, and volume to your calves. Since there are so many specific calf exercises I'll be using in this book, I've broken these down into the general body position needed when performing the necessary exercise movements. This way, when discussing exercises and routines in more detail, you'll have an idea of what's expected and how to get started.

1. **Standing calf exercises** – Standing calf exercises are calf raises performed in a standing position—on or off a machine, on one leg or two, and with or without weights. At the gym, do these exercises on a standing calf-raise machine, on a squat rack or Smith machine, with dumbbells or kettlebells, or on one leg or two. At home, you may or may not have similar equipment as at the gym, but you can

still perform standing calf exercises with or without weights, on the stairs, on steps, on the floor, or any elevated ledge that will support your weight. I'll discuss the many variations you can add throughout the rest of the book, to help you get the most out of your calf program.

2. **Seated calf exercises** – Seated calf raises are performed, as the name rightly suggests, while you are seated, generally using some form of equipment. Seated calf exercises can be performed with legs straight—on a leg press machine, or with legs bent—as with a seated calf machine. At the gym, seated calf exercises are generally performed with legs straight on a leg-press machine as an alternative or supplement to standing calf exercises because they also hit the gastrocnemius muscles. Seated calf exercises are performed on the seated calf machine with bent legs, with the exertion focusing on the soleus muscles. At home, assuming you don't have a leg press or seated calf-raise machine, seated calf exercises can be performed using a chair, with your legs bent and with weights resting on your knees and thighs, or while squatting with knees bent completely to mimic the seated calf-raise machine. Whether your legs are straight or bent, your calf exercises can be performed on one or two legs depending on how much weight or intensity you need. Almost any variation used with standing calf raises can be performed with seated calf raises.

3. **Calf exercises with a bent waist** – Calf exercises with a bent waist are generally performed either seated at the leg-press machine or standing with a bent waist for donkey calf raises. With seated calf raises on the leg press, the weight rests on your feet. In contrast, with donkey calf raises—

performed standing with a bent waist—the weight rests on your waist or lower back. Donkey calf raises can be performed on a donkey calf-raise machine, with weights hanging from around your waist, or with partners sitting on your lower back. At home, you will need to be creative to perform donkey calf raises and other standing bent waist calf exercise variations but suspending a weight from your waist will work if no family or friends volunteer to help.

4. **Dynamic calf exercises** – Although your body is moving during the other calf exercise positions, you are generally holding most of your body static through the exercises to focus the primary exertion within your calves. In contrast, dynamic calf exercises tend to be explosive and plyometric in nature, involving more of your body as you lift, jump, and exert powerfully, often leaving the ground as you thrust up or ahead. Jumping and sprinting exercises are typically the focus of dynamic calf exercises and range from jumping rope or jumping vertically in place, to plyometric leaps and hill sprints.

Although I've given a rough overview of calf-raise exercise types and the positions used in each category, there are many variations and options to add variety and intensity to these techniques. As you read, explore, and undertake your personal calf development journey, together we'll build on these foundational exercises throughout *Killer Calves*. The better your foundation, the better your calves.

EXERCISE VARIATIONS

Killer Calves is filled with different exercises and approaches to develop your calves. But one thing I need to stress is that you will ultimately have to find out what works best to achieve your calf goals. Whatever exercises and techniques you try, you will need to be persistent, maximize your effort, listen to your body, and, above all else, be willing to push your boundaries to achieve your dreams.

Every exercise routine in *Killer Calves* can be modified and adapted to help you grow and push your limits. Think of yourself as a mad fitness scientist searching out the best ways to unlock your growth potential. This process takes some work and quite a bit of creativity. Use this opportunity, your focused effort, and your ingenuity to your advantage to help yourself grow!

So, as you try out the routines and ideas in *Killer Calves*, here are some variations for almost any exercise to push your limits, overcome boredom and muscle adaptation, and build those calves! Ways to vary almost any exercise include:

1. **Reps** – Vary the number of repetitions required to push your limits. As your strength and endurance grow, increase the weight you push and/or the number of repetitions you perform.
2. **Sets** – Like reps, increasing or decreasing the numbers of sets by exercise type is always an option for calf development, whether your focus is on mass or definition.
3. **Time under tension** – Vary the time working, the time spent moving through the exercise, the time held contracting the calf at the top of the raise, and the time relaxed at the bottom of the motion to reduce or extend the time of your physical exertion.
4. **Weight** – Adding or subtracting weight is one of the classic ways to vary exercises. Not only can you add or subtract weight as you work through your sets, but you can also do the same within a set—drop sets or reverse drop sets. This will allow you to not only increase your total load—the amount of weight lifted in a given set—but can also extend your time under tension as you fight against muscle failure, such as when performing drop sets, to facilitate muscle growth.
5. **Explosivity** – Adjust the amount of energy or plyometric activation in each exercise. For instance, explode up during the calf raise and then lower slowly, or accelerate through your lift starting slowly and gradually building speed as you elevate.
6. **Change how you move through the exercise** – Employ continuous and discontinuous movements to shock your calves. For example, include pulses at the top of your calf raise while holding at full muscle extension and muscular concentration or include pauses or holds mid-motion.

7. **Exercise orientation** – Shift your foot orientation during the exercise. Classic examples include moving your toes out, pointing your toes in, or directing your toes forward during exercise.

8. **Change stress and strain direction** – Shift where the exercise tension moves through your calves by changing where the exertion moves through your feet when you push upward. For example, pushing up from and through your big toes instead of lifting from the balls of your feet or outside of them.

9. **Adjust the orientation of your bodyweight** – During exercise, adjust your body's angle to shift how the weight and exercise tension move through your muscles. For instance, lean forward, backward, sideways, or stay centered during the exercise to increase intensity and alter the focus of exertion.

10. **Adjust the smoothness or continuity of your motions** – Although you'll naturally tend to move fluidly through an exercise with continuity of motion, changing this will shock your muscles. Instead of completing the whole movement in one smooth motion, break it into sections.

11. **Surprise to overcome adaptation** – Change your routines to continue pushing your development. If your calves have adapted to your routine, their growth will suffer. A simple way to evaluate this is if they are no longer sore the day after your workout. If your calves aren't sore, consider changing your routine or increasing your workout intensity. If you haven't shocked your calves to the point of soreness, they are not going to respond with much growth.

12. **Electrical Muscle Stimulation (EMS)** – Stimulating your muscles with electrical impulses can certainly shock them

into growth. Some muscles respond more effectively than others to EMS training. In the case of calves, using EMS stimulation during your exercise routine, specifically in conjunction with weights and intense exertion, not only offers a novel way to train but can speed up results. In this instance, EMS can simulate adding additional weight and intensity to your calf routine without the risks of additional weight such as muscle tears, tendon damage, and joint pain. Consider EMS as another option to push yourself in new and growth-inducing ways.

13. **Combinations** – Any of these variations can be combined to add variety and increase effectiveness to your calf exercises, and, finally,

14. **Be original** – Think of your own variations to add to the list.

Variety is not only the spice of life; it is a key component of calf growth. Use these variations to keep your routines fresh and your calves growing!

Remember, this is a book about calf-building. So, although you often need to push your limits to get your calves to grow, you also need to be able to use them. Exercise intelligently and listen to your body to avoid injury. If you push yourself too hard, to the point of injury or inability to work out regularly, you won't be able to work those calves and your goals will suffer. Being out of action due to injury or discomfort for a few days is not going to help your calf growth goals, so take it steady and at an appropriate pace.

WAYS TO INCREASE YOUR CALVES' ABILITY TO GROW AND IMPROVE

Calves are stubborn. More than almost any other muscle group, they seem resistant to growth. To get your calves to respond, you need to find ways to overcome this resistance and increase their ability to respond to training.

Several factors can reduce or strongly influence your calves' potential to improve:

1. Your calves are highly adaptable muscles since you use them daily, even when not formally training.
2. Your calf anatomy—the attachment points of your calf muscle fibers on each leg, such as high versus low insertion points. High calf insertions reduce the overall growth area for the calf muscle while low calf insertions increase this area.
3. Failure to use proper form during exercise. Examples of improper form include using a short range of motion and

bouncing without proper muscle control through the movement. Improper form reduces time under tension, limiting muscle fiber engagement and growth potential.

4. Your calves have a very high elasticity or ability to stretch and rebound during exertion, allowing the calf muscle to extend more than two thirds of its range of motion and then recover quickly from tension transfer mediated by the Achilles tendon.

5. Your calf muscles' ratio of muscle fiber types—the percentage of fast versus slow twitch muscle fibers.

To maximize your growth potential, you need to attack and overcome the limiting factors you *can* control—your range of motion, muscle engagement, and time under tension.

To maximize your growth potential, for every repetition, increase the time under tension, maximize muscle engagement and exertion, put your awareness and focus into the muscle, and work to reduce the role of Achilles tendon elasticity during exercise—since the Achilles tendon reduces the calf muscles' contribution during each movement.

Combined, these approaches will ensure that the calf muscles do the majority of the work as you exercise. This means no bouncing, no partial reps, no releasing muscular tension, and no slacking... at least not until you've reached a point where you can't do much else or where exercises call for different techniques!

To help overcome these limitations, every single rep should be done with good form. Here's how. Consider this the foundational calf-raise form on which you'll build as your strength and experience grow:

1. Hold the stretch position—the lowest, fully extended position in most calf exercises—for at least two seconds to counter tendon elasticity, i.e. the Achilles tendon's capacity to stretch, transfer energy, and reduce full muscle engagement. Try to maintain tension in your hold—the stretch position is not a passive stretch and, to the extent possible, your muscles should be engaged.

2. Move slowly through the entire range of motion, especially the beginning of the reps, with control. Avoid accelerating and bouncing, so that you are controlling the weight and moving with purpose.

3. Hold the topmost contracted position—the highest, fully extended position in most calf exercises—for at least two seconds. Squeeze the muscle hard and put your mind—and your attention—into the muscle as you work.

4. Maintain maximum muscle tension as you lower the weight down. Resist the weight while you perform a controlled, negative exertion. You do not drop the weight down—you lower it through its full motion.

Calf growth routine:

Perform this superset to help boost your calf growth:

1. **Seated Calf Raises** – Using the principles of good form outlined above, perform 10-12 reps with no rest.

2. **Sled Pushing** – with a heavy load, push a weighted sled for 30 seconds.
3. **Rest** for 2 minutes. For best results, repeat the superset 2 to 3 more times.

With slow, controlled sets using maximal stretch and extension, full muscle engagement, and proper attention, your calves' ability to respond to training may surprise you.

BE THE CALF

Do your calves make chopsticks look thick?

The right program and frame of mind can fix that.

All you have to do is put your mind to it.

The secret to building phenomenal calves isn't about how much weight you can get them to move, although heavy weights *can* help. The secret to great calves is *being the calf*, feeling the calf muscles work through the entire range of exertion. Put your mind inside your muscles as you contract and relax.

Put your awareness in the muscles *throughout* your exercises.

But you're not just watching; you're engaging. This attention gets you to work, not watch. Use your awareness to enlist more muscle fibers, to stimulate the right muscles, to correct improper form, and to push harder and more completely than you would just counting reps or holding a position for some time.

Fully engaging in your exercises will not only focus your attention, but it will also stimulate your muscles through greater activation, help you observe opportunities for improvement, and spur your muscles on to greater growth.

Calves are no exception.

Use the following techniques to build your mind-muscle connection and encourage calf growth:

Seated Calf Flexes – Sit in a chair with your feet flat on the ground and legs bent at a 90-degree angle. Maintaining the seated, bent-legged position, lift up onto your toes one leg at a time. Hold this elevated position with your feet at full extension for 10 seconds. Contract your muscles, flexing as hard as you can while supporting your leg weight, then lower the foot and repeat, performing 3 to 4 calf flexes per side. The more seated calf flexes you perform each day, the better results you'll have.

Align Your Hips Properly – The angle of your hips plays a significant role in where you target your calf muscles, e.g., in the medial vs. lateral head muscles of the gastrocnemius. Involve the internal vs. external rotation angle of your hips in your calf training to find an angle that creates maximum calf muscle burn. Use the following steps to help adjust your hip alignment for targeted calf growth:

1. Start with your feet in a regular shoulder-width stance.
2. To focus on external hip rotation, keep your heels on the ground and rotate your toes away from one another, so that your heels are roughly shoulder-width apart while your toes shift out.

3. To focus on internal hip rotation, keep your toes on the ground and rotate your heels away from one another, so that your toes are roughly shoulder-width apart while your heels shift out.

4. For many people, the optimal angle will be about 45-degrees, but you will need to experiment to find what works best for you. Remember, you are looking for the angle that creates the most muscle burn. When performing targeted calf raises, do all your sets and reps at that angle.

Stand and Flex – Whenever you're standing in one place for extended periods, push up onto your toes using both calves, and flex. Hold this position until your calves start shaking, performing an extended isometric calf contraction. This isometric hold is perfect for when you're standing at your desk, standing by your counter cooking, working at a benchtop, or performing any other activity that gives the opportunity to carry out the exercise. Standing and flexing in place is also a great way to boost the mind-muscle connection with your calves—and your gains!

Every day is calf day – I mean it! Every time you work out, perform one set of calf exercises. Do this set on any suitable equipment using any calf-focused exercise, such as a standing calf-raise machine, a leg press, a seated calf-raise machine, a squat rack, or a donkey calf-raise machine. After warming up, do one pyramid set as below:

1. Using your chosen exercise, perform 10 reps using a full range of motion. Go as high onto your toes as you possibly

can on the last rep. Don't come down onto your heels after the last rep. Instead, do a 10-second isolation hold. Just hold that contraction at the top and squeeze hard. Put your mind —and effort—into the muscle.

2. Without rest, do another 10 reps. Go back into another 10-second isolation hold at full extension on the tips of your toes. As you fatigue, these may turn into partial reps. Fatigue and failure are okay; just don't give up.

3. Finally, to completely burn out your muscles, do another round of 10 reps and finish with one last 10-second isolation hold, going up onto your toes as high as possible. If your calves are not on fire and you can still perform complete reps by this point, you need to add more weight.

4. To help with recovery, immediately after the final isometric hold, lower your calves all the way down, and let the weight push down through your calves to stretch them. Hold this stretch for as long as possible. Alternate legs on the stretch as needed.

5. For the first week, do this program once per workout. After the first week, try to go through the workout twice. You might find it difficult to walk but your calves will grow.

The mind-muscle connection is exceptionally important for muscle growth. The mind-body connection, particularly learning to use this effectively, is also one of the weakest links in most people's overall fitness. Strengthen the mind-body link and your calves will have a shot at becoming the ideal you dream of every day.

TRAIN YOUR CALVES WITH STRAIGHT LEGS —A LITTLE CALF ANATOMY TO HELP YOUR MUSCLES GROW

Yes, your calves are stubborn, but, with a little understanding of *why* your calves aren't growing, you'll finally make them grow.

Your calves are comprised of three distinct muscle heads, the medial and lateral gastrocnemius, along with the underlying soleus.

While all three muscles have a distal attachment to the Achilles tendon that inserts onto the back of the heel, the proximal attachments are what separates the true calf muscles—the gastrocnemius—from the soleus.

The gastrocnemius are considered "dual joint" muscles because they cross two joints—the ankle and the knee. Most people don't understand this point, utilize this information, or effectively incorporate this understanding into their training.

In contrast to the gastrocnemius, the soleus muscle attaches onto the back side of the lower leg bones and never crosses the knee joint.

The soleus muscle only crosses the ankle joint.

This anatomical differentiation between the gastrocnemius and soleus muscles plays a major role in preventing people from building and developing their calf muscles.

Why does this anatomical difference matter?

Many people end up performing the calf raise movement incorrectly... at least for ideal muscle growth. Instead of stressing the gastrocnemius muscles, their training targets the stabilizer muscles of the lower leg, known as the soleus and medial flexor group.

With poor form, they miss out on fully engaging the two primary muscles in the calf that you want to grow to be aesthetically pleasing —to be ripped, full, huge, defined, or proportional to the rest of your body—the gastrocnemius.

To most effectively hit the gastrocnemius, ensure the knee is placed in a fully extended—straight—position when doing standing calf raises. The gastrocnemius muscles pass the knee joint and play a role in slight knee flexion. They also stabilize the knee. So, with this understanding in mind, the gastrocnemius *must* be trained with a straight-knee position to fully engage the calf muscles.

Most chicken-legged gym-goers do standing calf raises with slightly bent knees which shifts the emphasis to the soleus and flexors and elsewhere in the body, taking the weight away from the gastrocnemius.

So, the next time you're doing calf raises, especially while standing, use a full range of motion and make sure you maintain straight knees throughout the set.

You'll instantly feel the difference.

And your calves will thank you.

SLOW DOWN TO SPEED UP GAINS

Have you already tried standing calf raises with little success?

If so, you may be doing them incorrectly.

Your calves' weakness might come from one of your body's greatest strengths, your Achilles tendon, the thickest tendon in the body. The Achilles is meant for dynamic and explosive movements. So, whenever you hop on a standing calf-raise machine and bounce up and down banging out reps, your Achilles tendons have no problems managing that work, relieving the tension—and the workload— from the calves.

So, to see any gains, you have to target and isolate your calves during the workout.

To shift that work from the Achilles to the calves, you need to slow down and stop. Doing this as you perform your reps will remove as much of the Achilles' elastic stretch rebound as possible and focus on maximally lengthening and shortening your calf muscles. Slow down through the movement, pausing while fully extended for most benefit. Combining this controlled movement with straight legs—in standing calf raises—will also prevent the tension from moving away from the gastrocnemius and into other leg areas.

Here's how to perform calf raises with a minimum 8-second pause in your reps to unlock their growth potential:

1. Hold the stretch position—the bottom position of your calf raises with your heels lowered as much as possible—for 5 seconds on every rep.
2. With your knees straight—to keep the tension on your calves and not elsewhere in your legs—push up slowly, controlling the weight with your exertion.
3. Hold the contracted position—the top position at full extension—for at least 3 seconds on every rep.
4. Lower slowly, engaging your muscles as you drop, then repeat.
5. Perform 4 sets of 12 reps in each set, rotating through different calf exercise variations each time you work them, such as changing toe positions.
6. Carry out this calf routine at least twice a week. As you get stronger, add more weight and/or increase the time taken for each repetition of the calf raise. You could also hold your contractions and stretches for longer.

If you've been bouncing when working your calves, then the difference in feeling your muscles actually work will be striking. Also, because you'll be working your calves instead of your tendons, be prepared for more muscle soreness. As an added bonus, the extended time held in the stretch position during calf raises will also help to stretch out your Achilles tendons if they're tight.

And remember, when training your calves, slow, controlled motions speed up gains.

VARIETY IS THE SPICE OF LIFE...FOR CALF GAINS

Don't blame your genetics for your weak lower legs. Blame your training—or its absence. Many weightlifters' calf workouts involve rapid, shallow reps... that's if they do any training for calves at all, of course.

When you exercise, don't be a calf bouncer or bobber. Getting your calves to grow requires loaded flexion and extension of the ankles. Most people neglect this important point and miss a significant side benefit of calf training: strong feet and ankles.

Poor exercise mechanics doesn't just hurt your calf gains though.

Poor mechanics when exercising your calves ultimately affects your gains and performance of other important lifts too.

Here are some tools to strengthen your feet, improve your ankle mobility, help your calves grow bigger, and improve the entire foundation of your lower-body training to help you squat, deadlift, press, and grow with the best of them.

. . .

Paused Calf Raises - If you are like most gym goers, you've probably been doing calf raises as though you're bouncing on a trampoline. While this may make you think you're working out your calves as you throw around heavy weights, you're really just putting your Achilles tendons through their paces. Don't fool yourself. Bouncy, shallow reps are not the way to get your calves to grow.

Athletes depend on the elastic nature of the Achilles tendon for jumping, running, and rapid movement shifts. But Achilles training will not build your calves. Look no further than the kangaroo. What has elastic bouncing done for kangaroos' calves? If you want kangaroo calves, however, bounce away.

If you allow elastic, springy movements to predominate in your calf training, you'll reduce the effectiveness of your calf exercises. Pausing at the top and bottom on any calf raise will limit the Achilles tendon's involvement in the exercise. Without this elastic contribution, your calf muscles will do more work. More work equals more growth. More control equals less Achilles involvement.

When performing your calf raises, pause at the top and bottom of the motion for at least two seconds. Stretch the calf at the bottom as much as possible without pain by allowing your heels to drop and your toes to point upward. Then, after this pause, push as high as possible onto the balls of your feet and toes. Hold your calf raise again at the top of the lift.

If you want to develop better strength and mobility at the end of your exertion ranges in your calf exercises—under full downward stretch and upward contraction in the hold positions at the top and bottom of the rep—you should work on controlling the exercise movements under load at the tops and bottoms of your lifts. As you gain more control in the tops and bottoms of your lifts, your ankles and feet will grow stronger. Take a similar approach to reap benefits in other exercises as well, such as squatting, benching, curls, or any other exercise.

To start, choose a load you're able to control and press with full ankle dorsiflexion and extension or you'll default to bouncing the weight. Allow yourself to settle into the stretch using the weight as a guide. Use a similar approach to your other calf-raise variations.

If your calves are tight and prevent you getting a full stretch at the bottom of your exercise, then try foam rolling to release the muscles. Alternate between foam rolling your calves for 10 rolls and static stretching them for 20-30 seconds each. Repeat 2 to 3 times and then try flexing your ankles. Be persistent and keep stretching over time to help get your flexibility where it's needed. If you have damaged your ankles from past injuries and have ankle sprains and strains, for example, then stretching becomes very important to overcome potential movement limitations.

Also, be sure to vary your rep ranges and train your calves frequently. Our calves evolved to let us stand and walk on them all day and each day. Doing 3 to 4 sets of 8-10 reps once a week won't shock your muscle into growth.

Tiptoe Farmer's Carries - Farmers, used to physical labor, are often far stronger than you might guess, especially based on appearances. Hauling around heavy objects such as sacks of feed, machine parts, and other necessities daily is part of the reason they're so strong. Use the farmer's secret weapon—lifting heavy stuff as you move—as a key to calf development.

To get started, pick up suitable weights—the heavier the better—and walk on your tiptoes across the gym, your living room, or wherever you're working out. Don't worry about any strange looks you may receive as you move around; those looks will turn to envy as your calves grow. Channel your inner farmer or strongman as you lug around those dumbbells. Use the tiptoe farmer carry as a more effective alternative to the seated calf machine.

Tip: Use a weight that allows you to maintain full ankle plantar flexion—a full extension onto the balls of your feet, extending up onto your tiptoes as you stand. This will strengthen your feet, help develop ankle control, and smash your calves.

Single-Leg Kettlebell Passes - One of the most effective ways to strengthen your ankles, feet, and calves is to do challenging single-leg exercises. Examples include single-leg squats, split-squat variations, and single-leg deadlifts. As you balance on them, the muscles in your feet and ankles work harder because you engage stability muscles. This balancing act also makes you focus your attention on the muscles working to keep you stable, creating a forced mind-muscle connection. Stronger feet and ankles play a key role in your ability to handle heavier weights and in getting your calves to grow.

Challenge your arches and ankles with this simple drill. Stronger arches and ankles are especially valuable for those who overpronate or have flat feet.

Stand on one leg holding a kettlebell in one hand at your side. While maintaining balance on one foot, slowly pass the kettlebell across your body and over to the opposing hand. You can also perform this exercise with a dumbbell, but, given its ergonomics, a kettlebell is easier to pass between hands. Slowly pass the kettlebell to the opposite hip, hold for a moment, and then reverse the movement. Pass the kettlebell back and forth for 4 to 6 passes for 2 to 3 sets on each leg. Progressive loading matters less than maintaining control and balance in the exercise.

• • •

Sled Pushes - Many people think of sleds as a tool for conditioning, athletic training, or for hauling presents at Christmas. But the sled also works for those seeking bigger, stronger physiques—especially calves and legs—and a better overall work capacity.

Sled pushing is concentric-focused, so the exercise doesn't cause serious soreness like some other calf exercises. Sled pushing is a safe, effective way to load and train your calves and ankles in the way they're meant to move. To top off your overall gains, sled pushing engages your glutes and quads in addition to your calves, adding a variety of benefits to your routine.

As you perform the exercise, take natural, deliberate strides while you push a loaded sled over 20 to 50 yards or meters of turf. Maintain tension in your abdominal muscles for stability and keep a natural, neutral spine as you move your hips with each stride. As you work, use the ground to push the sled forward, connecting solidly through your feet. Load the sled with additional weight to do some serious exercise.

Perform 3 to 4 sets of sled pushes after any workout for some high-intensity anaerobic interval training.

Calf training doesn't have to be a chore.

Use the exercises in *Killer Calves* to not only improve your calf development and overcome plateaus but to keep your workouts fun and enjoyable.

Remember, the more you enjoy your workouts, the more likely you are to do them on a regular basis. And regular, dedicated exercise is a vital key to calf growth.

CALF ROUTINES OF THE HUGE AND FAMOUS

Many people are famous for their physiques, just as there are many who are famous for their knowledge. There are also some who are famous for their calves.

Here, I'll spread a bit of these calf legends' knowledge so that you can enjoy their phenomenal physiques.

Arnold Schwarzenegger's Conan Calves[1]

Arnold is a true legend, and so are his calves. Arnold, among many other things, is famous for transforming his calves from tiny saplings into mighty oaks.

Here are a couple of Arnold's routines:

· · ·

Arnold's Calf Routine 1:

Exercise	Sets	Reps
Monday / Wednesday / Friday		
Donkey Calf Raises	4	10
Standing Calf Raises	4	10
Seated Calf Raises	4	10
Tuesday / Thursday / Saturday		
Standing Calf Raises	4	15, 10, 8, 8
Calf Raises on a Leg-Press Machine	4	10

Arnold believes in the benefits of volume training with high training loads to stimulate muscle growth, and this routine reflects these volume-based beliefs. This program also shows how much Arnold believes in and dedicates to working his calves. This routine requires being totally committed to your calf development, and in the gym six days a week. As in many of Arnold's routines, his programs are a gold standard of fitness—well thought out, proven, comprehensive, and results-driven.

Arnold's Calf Routine 2:

Donkey Calf Raise - Sets: 5-6, Reps: 15-20.
Standing Calf Raise - Sets: 5-6, Reps: 10-20.
Seated Calf Raise - Sets: 4-5, Reps: 10-15.

Arnold's advice on calf training in his own words:

• • •

"The main exercises I did shouldn't surprise you: donkey calf raises, standing calf raises, seated calf raises, and leg press calf raises—up to six sets of each for 10–20 reps. But more important than the exercise I was doing, or the number of sets and reps I performed, was how I did them.

"To develop your calves to their potential, you must take each rep through a complete range of motion. This means getting a full stretch at the bottom and forcing yourself up as high as possible on your toes at the top. Again, it's about progression; if you're using 1,000 pounds but can't go all the way up, you're training too heavy and wasting your time. The goal is to lift the heaviest weight possible that still allows you to use a full range of motion.

"I also used other techniques to squeeze out every last bit of intensity and spark new growth. Other than doing forced reps with the help of a partner, my favorite techniques were peak contractions and what I used to call a 'pumping action'.

"Peak contraction is simply a matter of holding the top of each rep and squeezing the calves for three to four counts before lowering the weight. This was very painful, but I always relished the muscle burn and felt it would only make me bigger. The pumping action would usually take place at the end of a set of, say, seated calf raises or leg press calf raises. After I couldn't do any more full-range-of-motion reps, I finished the set by doing short, quick reps (not quite all the way up or down) for as long as possible until my calves were screaming. I felt this action really chiseled the outer section of my calves for championship form."

Lou Ferrigno's Hulk Calves[2]

. . .

Being the Incredible Hulk wasn't the only thing incredible about Lou Ferrigno. His calves are pretty incredible as well. Use this routine to hulk out your own calves too.

Lou's Calf Routine:

Standing Calf Raise - Sets: 10-12, Reps: 6-10.
Seated Calf Raise - Sets: 10-12, Reps: 15-20.

Lou's advice on calf training in his own words:

"I like to devote one calf workout to the soleus muscle with seated calf raises (10 to 12 sets of 6 to 10 reps) and the next calf workout to the gastrocnemius with standing calf raises (10 to 12 sets of 15 to 20 reps)."

Tom Platz's Mega Calves[3]

Tom Platz is known for having some of the best legs of his generation, and any other. Although many remember his thighs, Tom's calves were the foundation upon which his phenomenal legs were built.

While Arnold is known for his preference for donkey calf raises, Tom preferred the static rep—holding a very heavy weight at full or partial extension—to help stimulate calf growth.

. . .

Tom's Calf Routine:

Standing Calf Raises - Sets: 3-4, Reps: 10-15.
Seated Calf Raises - Sets: 3-4, Reps: 10-15.
Hack Machine Calf Raises - Sets: 3-4, Reps: 10-15.
Static Calf Holds - Hold your maximum weight at full extension for as long as possible (e.g. seated on a leg press machine).

Tom's calf training in his own words:

"I'm going to tell you some stuff that I never really tell most people.

"Back in my day, everybody did calves like six days a week, but I had most success training calves twice a week. With my body type, really intense calf training twice a week proved to be most effective.

"I did normal calf raises, standing calf raises, seated calf raises primarily, those two major exercises. The one thing I did on the standing calf raise on certain days, and on the seated calf raise, at the end of my workout, I would put slowly and progressively, as many plates as possible. Joe Gold made a special seated calf machine, extended the bar so I could put ten 100-pound plates or fifteen 100-pound plates. My goal was to just hold the weight at the end of my workout. Many workouts I would just hold the weight, not up high, not real low, but in the middle. I would just hold it. Imagine just holding 1000 or 2000 pounds at the end of your routine, just holding it still until I could barely hold it.

"I'd have some of the monster guys in the gym push on it barely, watch me, stay close to me. As soon as I felt like it was getting too much and my tendons and ligaments couldn't handle the tension, I would say, "Take it now!" and they took it.

"My message to you is that the static rep, the partial static rep, maybe once a week, maybe twice a week at the most, proved to be unbelievable, magic for my calves. I never wanted to get implants. Between getting implants or doing heavy static partial work, the heavy training, hard work, old school training methodology worked best. That's the actual fact. I don't think I ever said that to a writer in a magazine. I may have. That works best for calves for me. One day I would do higher reps prior to that, of course, one day I did real low reps, and I alternated that. But, always, static reps proved to be most effective."

Erik Fankhouser's Mountainous Calves[4]

Erik has legendary calves. Unlike Arnold, Erik won the calf genetics lottery. But that hasn't stopped Erik from pushing his calves to their limits to achieve legendary gains.

Erik's Calf Routine:

Week 1:

Seated Calf Raise - Sets: 4, Reps: 12.

Leg Press Calf Raise - Sets: 4, Reps: 12.
Reverse Calf Raise - Sets: 4, Reps: 12.

Week 2:

One-leg Smith Machine Standing Calf Raise - Sets: 4, Reps: 15.
One-leg Donkey Calf Raise - Sets: 4, Reps: 15.
One-leg Reverse Calf Raise - Sets: 4, Reps: 15.

Erik's calf training in his own words:

"Yes, I've always had good calf development. I always tell people that I was 150 pounds and my calves were as big as they are now. They obviously weren't, but they were always pretty freaky. I had football-sized calves when I was in middle school. I've definitely brought them up through training, but at this point I'm not trying to add any more mass; just stimulate them to maintain what I have. They are my money-maker, so I have to keep them there."

James "Flex" Lewis's Superhero Calves[5]

. . .

Flex's calves are so impressive, he actually has to moderate his training to keep his body in balance. Here's an overview of one of Flex's calf training routines so you too can have monster calves.

Flex is an innovator who is constantly pushing himself with high-intensity training, coming up with new exercise variations and challenges, adapting to his needs while pushing his limits. His great calves are a result of these intensely dynamic efforts.

Lewis says, "My calf training is crazy."

After trying his workout, you'll see why.

Flex's Calf Routine:

Exercise	Sets	Reps
Leg press calf raises	4	25-35
Seated calf raises	4	25-35
Standing calf raises	3	25-35

Calf training tips from Flex:

- Before starting calf exercises, warm up and stretch your legs fully.
- Perform your reps quickly, the more the better. Weight is not the main consideration when training calves. The goal of the calf routine is to keep your blood flowing throughout the calf muscles while exercising.
- When training calves, find the optimal rhythm, timing, variations, and mix of movements to amplify your routine and development.
- Make sure your legs are fully pumped before stopping your calf routine. If your legs are too fatigued to do more reps with weight, use bodyweight calf raises to finish your calf workout.

Training calves with dedication has helped make the careers—and bodies—of the world's most elite bodybuilders. Even if you're not a bodybuilder, take the advice of some of the world's best bodybuilders to get your calves to grow!

CALF RAISES WITH STIFF-LEGGED JUMPS

Being intelligent about how you attack your calves is critical in capturing the muscle development you're after. Recognizing your calves are made up of different muscle groups and muscle fiber types, each which responds more readily to different stimuli, is critical to getting your calves to grow.

Use this dynamic superset to work your calves' slow and fast-twitch muscle fibers, hitting the muscles from different angles and speeds to shock them into growth:

1. **Standing Calf Raises** - Start this routine at the standing calf-raise machine. Do eight full, controlled reps. Make sure to pause for two-seconds at the bottom of each rep. Try to rest no longer than 10 to 15 seconds before moving on to the next movement. Having your barbell loaded and ready for your upcoming calf jumps will allow you to control rest times and keep your exercise tempo high.

2. **Weighted Calf Jumps** - Add roughly 25% of your body weight onto a barbell. Hold the loaded bar resting on your shoulders in a standing position as you would at the start of a squat and, with minimal knee bend and a neutral spine, jump up and down, pushing up and through with the calves on each rep. Fully extend your toes downward as you jump upward to maximize your calves' engagement. Target 30 reps to start. The eccentric loading caused by the jumping and landing will encourage muscle growth.

3. **Repeat** - Perform the calf raise / calf jump superset combination four more times for five total sets.

As your strength improves, consider increasing the weight you use, the volume of your jumps, the height and intensity of your jumps, and the number of sets performed.

For variety, take your calf jumps outside using dumbbells or a weighted vest while performing single-leg calf raises on stairs or a curb. The ground, especially a grassed field, will be more forgiving on your joints.

The combination of calf raises and calf jumps should spur your calf growth to new heights.

STAIRWAY TO CALVES

The world is full of opportunities to build your calves. In writing *Killer Calves*, I hope to help you learn to see these opportunities too, and come up with many new growth-inducing variations that I haven't discovered. And—thankfully for your calves and the potential to help them grow—the world is also full of stairs.

Using stairs to help your calves grow is simple. Here's how you do it:

1. **Find suitable stairs**. If you don't have access to stairs, use a rock, a curb, or find a stable rectangular block… nothing should stop you from reaching your calf goals!
2. **Perform one-legged calf raises on the stairs using your bodyweight only.** Hold the stretch position for five seconds on every rep. Do five reps, then switch legs.

3. **Repeat.** Go up to the next step and perform single-leg calf
   raises for each leg.

Note: Try to find a set of stairs to do at least 50 reps per calf in a
sequence, climbing up one step at a time after finishing each set with
both legs. Going up one step at a time helps with your counting.
That's 10 stairs at a minimum. There are no excuses... not even
having no stairs!

Make this routine a habit and your calves will thank you for it.

If you have stairs in your house, do this twice a day.

If you don't have stairs, find an alternative.

Be warned, don't go crazy at first trying to build your calves using
the stairs. Unless you've been working consistently with calf training,
the soreness can be debilitating. You won't be able to walk or workout
properly. And that will hurt your gains!

See the *Variations* chapter for more ways to push this program.

Consider anything from:

1. **Adding weights** - A weight vest works nicely to increase
   your workout's intensity while keeping the additional
   weight load aligned with your body structure throughout
   the movement.
2. **Increasing the number of stairs climbed** - More steps
   increases the number of sets performed.
3. **Increasing the number of reps performed on each step** -
   For example, doing 10 reps per leg instead of 5.

4. **Changing the timing or tempo of your reps** - Extending the stretch at the bottom of the rep and/or the contraction/hold at the top of the exertion. For example, a 5 or 10-second stretch or contraction held at full extension.

5. **Get creative!** - There are many other options to overcome your body's ability to adapt, from changing tempo, body orientation, and adding pauses mid-rep.

For example, one of my favorite variations is performing each rep with a 5 second contraction while wearing a weight vest. Maintaining the 50 total repetition target, do sets of 10 on each step finishing on the fifth step or keep pushing beyond 50 total reps. For additional fun—pain—hold your final contraction for as long as possible, such as a twenty count or whatever brings the burn. While doing this final contracted hold, lift up as high onto your toes as possible.

Remember, pushing yourself and your limits helps your calves grow!

MAXIMIZE TIME UNDER TENSION FOR CALF GAINS

Maximizing time under tension, the amount of time you are exerting during exercise, is a key ingredient to significant calf gains.

Calves can be a very challenging—and by challenging I mean frustrating—muscle group. If they don't have well-developed calves naturally, many people have to work their tails off to get them.

If you're reading this book, you're probably one of those hard gainers. To overcome the calf growth challenge, you need to combine quite a few factors to get the most effective stimulation.

Here are a few ways to build your calves by focusing on increased time under tension (the time spent working during sustained exertion without rest or recovery):

1. **Work your calves by combining heavy weights and high**

reps with very short rest periods between sets. Perform calf circuits using different exercise angles to hit the muscles from various directions but be sure to keep the weights heavy and the reps high. For variations, add some tempo manipulation by moving fast or slow through the exercise as well as adding pauses at your peak contraction and stretched position. Just because you've failed performing the full range of motion does not mean you cannot perform a portion of the exercise via a partial rep. Adding pulses at peak contraction after you can no longer push through the full exercise range will push your time under tension and help stimulate calf growth.

2. **Find a Smith machine and use it!** Perform Smith machine standing barbell calf raises. The stability-providing support posts from the Smith machine will let you lift heavy weights without losing movement quality from trying to balance the weight on your shoulders. Perform 12-15 reps per set to start. Hold a three-second pause at the peak calf contraction and a three-second pause at the stretch during the first or second half of your set for a simple exercise variation. Pause times can be changed based on weight used and your fitness level to maximize time under tension.

3. **Get creative with gym equipment.** Perform one-legged calf raises on the leg-press machine. Start with 12-15 reps per set. During the first half of the set, use a full range of motion using a complete stretch and toe extension as you push the weight. On the last half of the set, use partial extensions focusing on the top half of the movement. As with the Smith machine calf raises above, or when using other techniques from the *Variations* chapter, consider

varying your exercise tempo to optimize your muscles' time under tension.

4. **Get off your feet, but don't rest!** Instead, go find a seated calf machine. Perform heavy seated calf raises to failure. Use variations discussed above including pulses, pauses and holds, adjusting the tempo of your lift, drop sets, and using various angles to hit the muscles from different sides.

5. **Sprint.** Sprinting is a great way to push your time under tension, especially as part of a larger calf program. After warming up, sprint 40 to 60 yards or meters, repeating your sprints 6 to 8 times. Sprint as fast as possible and then jog back to your starting point. Sprint twice per week and focus on running on the balls of your feet as you go. Sprinting up hills makes the pain and growth even better. Vary your speed, distance, and rest times to add variety. See the chapter on sprinting and hill running for more ideas.

6. **Walk.** Yes, walk. Find the steepest hill you can. If you don't have a hill, use a treadmill set at the maximum incline setting, or simply use stairs. Walk briskly, as fast as possible, up the hill. Concentrate on engaging your calves as you walk and move through a complete range of motion with each step. Vary your tempo, going 20 to 30 seconds as fast as possible, then walk at a normal pace for the same amount of time. Add a backpack or weighted vest to push you during your hill or incline walks. Incorporate plyometric movements like skips and jumps for variation. Imagine you're hiking up a beautiful mountain to help those calves grow. The view from the top will be worth it!

To maximize your calf gains, you have to be willing to push them creatively. Whether that is through long, intense or frequent sets, while employing exercise variations in both, is up to you. As long as you give your body enough time to recover and avoid injury between sessions, maximizing time under tension is a surefire path to calf growth.

CALF RAISE AWAY TO BRING THE GAINS ALL DAY

Since calf muscles often respond well to exercises involving higher numbers of repetitions—due to their muscle fiber make-up and high physiologic stress tolerance—this high frequency training (HFT) program can help you improve your calf strength and enjoy more calf growth than you ever have before.

More than just an exercise routine to be done when you work out, think of this program as a slight lifestyle change, one in which you incorporate calf training daily. If you've already committed to exercising regularly, this routine is merely a calf-focused extension to that commitment.

High frequency single-leg calf raise program:

How Strong Are You? Before you begin this program, you need to determine your initial strength level. This evaluation requires an honest assessment of your initial strength. Since this is about you and you alone, do not cheat! You're performing this program for your betterment, not your ego. No one needs to know your results and you're not comparing yourself to anyone.

Calf Strength Test (Baseline strength):

To start, without shoes, perform one set of single-leg calf raises with each leg.

If at first the bare floor is too hard on your feet, carpet is fine, but you should work toward being comfortable on all surfaces.

Use as little assistance as possible to maintain your balance while performing your calf raises.

Use just your fingertips resting lightly on a countertop or against a wall to maintain your balance.

Try to perform 3 to 4 single-leg calf raises without holding onto anything to engage your ankle stabilizers to get a sense of the motion —the balance and stability required for the unassisted single-leg calf raises.

Take a short break and then see how many unassisted single-leg calf raises you can do with each leg. Go for it!

Tips:

1. Keep your exercising leg completely straight during every repetition to only engage your calf muscles. There should be no swaying or pumping via torso shifting or knee flexion to facilitate the calf raise.
2. Keep your body in a proper, vertical alignment while you lift.

3. Again, you are not trying to impress anyone, just to better yourself in the privacy of your own home or anywhere else you choose. This honest baseline assessment will show you how much opportunity you have to improve your functional strength and calf growth.
4. Note how many reps you perform with each leg. The goal here is at least 20 good clean reps, your baseline strength for each leg.

The Routine - This high-frequency training routine is the heart of the program, the one that will boost your strength and your calves with it.

Perform 3 sets of single-leg calf raises with as many reps as possible (AMRAP) with each leg every day, at morning, midday, and night using the techniques outlined in the initial strength test, such as straight legs, no skipping/cheating, and minimal support. Push yourself to see those results! Technique tips:

Begin with your stronger calf to help create your target goals, as you want each calf as strong as the other, establishing neural carryover to your weaker side, making you stronger and more goal focused.

Perform each calf raise slowly. Drive up through the ball of your foot onto your big toe and reach the highest elevation possible by squeezing your calf muscle to peak tension. Hold the raise at full extension for 2 seconds with each rep.

Maintain good posture via a long, relaxed spine, to help facilitate proper form and reduce risks of cramping while exercising.

Spread the sets evenly throughout the day. Perform one set in the morning, one in the afternoon, and one in the evening. There is no break for great calves!

Do not perform any additional calf training in your normal workouts.

Perform the sets barefoot to maximally engage your calves through a complete range of motion. You can wear shoes of course. Just make sure to get all your sets in, whether at work, home, or wherever possible.

Stop your set once your knee flexes, you can no longer stabilize, or your ability to elevate onto your toes decreases by one inch (two centimeters).

Rest for 30 seconds between each side.

Do this routine every day for two weeks.

The Retest - You've committed to your calves for two weeks. Now you get to see how far you've come!

After 2 weeks of daily calf training, the time has come to retest your standing, single-leg calf raise performance.

Before testing, take one full day off from calf raises.

The following day, after 48 hours from your last set of calf raises, retest your standing single-leg calf raise following the guidelines above—good form, maintain body alignment, and no cheating—with **one** exception. Do not include the 2-second peak contraction in the test sets. Otherwise, perform a normal set of as many reps as possible.

If you still fall short of the 20-repetition target, continue with the daily program for two more weeks and retest again.

Depending on your performance, keep extending the program until you reach your goal, if you achieve the goal with one leg but not the other.

• • •

Keep Pushing! - You are not done! There are many more goals and variations ahead if you decide to keep pushing and improving in your single-leg calf training.

New targets:

You could work toward performing standing single-leg calf raises *without any* balance assistance.

You could work toward performing unassisted single-leg calf raises with your opposite knee raised up, your opposite leg forward, backward, or out to the side.

You could incorporate this program into your exercise routine indefinitely to keep pushing those gains.

Use variations to increase your limits, increase your strength, and boost your growth further.

While exercises with strict form are a great place to start your single-leg program, variations can help push your improvements over the top. Options include:

1. Pulsing at the top of your contraction motion after reaching the point where you can no longer perform full reps, to maximize the burn and muscle fatigue.
2. Destabilizing your body by leaning slightly forward or backward to force your muscles to fire and contract in new ways as you perform reps.
3. Slowing down the contraction (lifting) and relaxation (lowering) sections of your calf raises.
4. Holding the peak contraction for longer than 2 seconds.
5. Adding weight while maintaining strict form.
6. Never letting your heel touch the ground to maintain tension throughout each set.
7. Incorporating any other suggestions mentioned in the *Variations* chapter.

If you question that a seemingly simple program like this one works, just look at the calf development of almost any ballet dancer. You'll see real-world proof that unassisted calf raises on the floor, lifting consistently at high volume, will do wonders for your calf development.

Once you're able to perform 10 perfect, single-leg calf raises unassisted while holding a 2-second peak contraction at the top of each rep, you will achieve an above average level of calf size and strength. From there, using the continued supplemental options outlined above, you can leave *normal* far behind.

THE DANCER'S CALF-TRAINING ANSWER

If you look across all athletic groups as a whole and evaluate them by calf aesthetics—particularly relative to body size and shape—to determine which group has the best calves, you would be hard-pressed to find a group with better calves than dancers.

Good cases for the best athletes' calves could also be made for sprinters—track and field and cycling—and gymnasts.

Dancers, too, have amazing calves. When you compare dancers' calves against those of many gym-goers, you will agree that the dancers' greatest strength is many gym-goers' most glaring weakness.

So, if you've tried almost every calf-training approach known to both man and gym monsters—drop sets, reverse drop sets, plyometrics, negative-accentuated/eccentric training, explosive movements/concentric training, extended sets, isometrics, tempo adjustments, extended burns, supersets, tri-sets and giant sets, escalating density training, partial reps, training with perfect form, unilateral training, stair climbing, hill sprints, high-intensity interval training, farmer's carries, and any other program or idea the gym gods can summon—you may want to consider training your calves like a dancer.

You can still train the rest of your body like the Incredible Hulk but take your calf cues from the amazing legs of dancers. Then your whole body will hulk out.

Dancer's Calves

Dancers are constantly using their calves, consistently and repetitively up on their toes, holding their calves contracted at full extension while balancing on the balls of their feet. They are jumping explosively over and over while focusing the effort into their calves. and moving up and down with precision as well as explosion. Dancers, as much as any athlete, are performing more bodyweight calf raises than just about anyone else.

In ballet, lifting up onto your toes using bodyweight calf raises is known as relevé. For you, lifting up onto your toes is called calf gains.

I'm are not asking you to wear a tutu—though you can if you so wish—but I am asking you to consider calf training like someone who wears a tutu. If you want to experience the calf hypertrophy effects of a dancer, and enjoy their excellent calf development, then start your dancer training today.

The solution is simple: perform at least 100 reps of daily bodyweight calf raises. As with the three-times-a-day single-leg calf-training program from the last chapter, the dancer's calf program can be considered a lifestyle choice incorporated into your daily routines.

Do this dancer's calf program every day and watch your spindly chopsticks transform into tree trunks.

. . .

The Dancer's Calf Program:

Standing calf raises on the floor:

Begin your dancer's calf program by performing 50 repetitions of calf raises from the floor.

The goal is to work up to at least 100 reps using only your bodyweight.

Perform this workout religiously every day for a month. Not only will your calves grow but also, your balance and coordination will improve.

Proper form when performing your standing calf raises is very important.

Stand with your feet roughly shoulder-width apart, angling your toes slightly outward. Concentrate on raising your heels straight upward without flexing your knees or bouncing your body up and down as you lift. As you exert, try to isolate as much tension into your calves as possible. This is how your calves grow!

Contract your calves hard at the top of each exertion. Try not to hold onto anything for support. This will only limit your load and your gains with it. Avoiding assistance will also make sure your stabilizing muscles are fully engaged and become stronger. To limit assistance and involve stabilizing muscles, let your arms relax by your sides or place your hands on your hips. If you need to hold your arms up or out to assist with balance, that is fine.

Perform the exercises in bare feet without shoes. This will allow a greater range of motion and force you to involve more muscles as you work. Raise your heels as high as possible off the ground. Be sure to distribute your weight evenly over the entirety of the balls of your feet and toes. Hold the top contraction at full extension for at least 2 seconds. Do not cheat or bounce! You must pause, coming to a defined stop at the peak contraction. You *must* feel a contraction in the calves as you hold at the top of the exercise.

Lower slowly in a controlled fashion. Don't just plop back to the ground as though you're falling onto the couch after work. If you don't raise and lower correctly, the rep doesn't count. These calf raises have to be quality repetitions to get the most from this type of training—quality reps with quality form = gains. Not only will your primary gastrocnemius calf muscles burn, but so will your stabilizing muscles as well. Hitting all these muscles will make huge differences to your calf development.

This program will take about 10 minutes a day over a month to start seeing results. Each controlled repetition will take about 6 seconds in total, 2 seconds to raise, 2 seconds held at the peak contraction, and 2 seconds to lower with no pause at the bottom. Since you'll be performing roughly 100 reps per day, you'll be working your calves for about 10 minutes daily. Throw in stretching and any cooldown and you'll add another minute or more. A small sacrifice with proven results.

Aside from getting massive calves, this program has the benefit of being doable anywhere at any time. No special equipment or memberships are required. All that is needed is your commitment and effort to see great gains.

Keep working and challenging yourself until you reach a level of calf development you're satisfied with relative to your goals. Then consider reducing your workload to 2 to 3 sessions a week to maintain those gains or keep pushing for more. If you return to using other equipment for your calves, just one session a week should help maintain your new development and give you a break from potential boredom. For other bonus options to keep those challenges and gains coming, see below.

Bonus Work for Bonus Gains:

Once you have completed your first full month of the dancer calf program, add an additional 5, 10, or 20 pounds using a weighted vest, dumbbell, kettlebell, or plate, and go at it again. If the standing calf raises are too easy for you at any time, think about adding additional weight earlier in the program.

Use other variations in addition to, or as an alternative to, more weight. For example, add a longer peak contraction at the top of your raise, slow the rate you lift and lower your body, lift your arms overhead to change the balance component, or increase the number of repetitions performed.

Be prepared to work through the burn. Once you come out of the fire on the other side, your calves will thank you.

And even dancers will be envious.

HIT THE HILLS FOR GREAT CALVES (AND LEGS)

The hills are alive with calves!

If you want to build calf muscles quickly, hill sprints are a great way to go.

To start, find a hill that is about 50 to 200 yards or meters long. If you live in an area that is relatively flat and doesn't have any suitable hills, use a treadmill set on a steep incline over the same distance for similar results. Stairs are also an option as long as there are enough flights to challenge you.

Take time to warm up sufficiently before starting your hill routine —your hamstrings, muscles, and tendons will all benefit. Whether that's walking and jogging up the hill or around the area, dynamic stretching, jumping jacks, or running in place, be prepared for the amount of difficult exertion required by hill running.

Hill Running Overview:

.   .   .

Now that you've found a suitable hill and have warmed up, sprint up the hill close to your maximum speed and strength. When running, be sure you're moving through full extension with your feet to fully activate the calves. Run in a natural upright posture, keeping your neck, back, and shoulders relaxed, trying not to lean forward into the hill. When you reach the top of the hill, let your momentum continue for a few yards or meters, relaxing and letting the tension out of your muscles as you slow down.

Then, jog back down the hill.

Repeat the drill 5 to 10 times, or more if you're ready and want to push yourself.

As you become more comfortable with hill running, bump up the intensity and volume and add in more variations.

Complete Basic Sprint Workout with Warmup:

Directions: With dynamic stretching—active movements where your joints and muscles go through a full range of motion to prepare for exertion—perform each moving 'stretch' for at least two seconds (e.g. legs swings, hip circles, arm circles, torso twists, walking knee to chest raises, straight leg kicks, etc. should each last a couple of seconds as you move dynamically through the stretch), and repeat each dynamic movement to get your body ready. When sprinting, your rests and recovery periods are between each sprint, and determined by how long you take to jog or walk back down the hill. But remember, don't draw your breaks out too much.

Warmup:

1. **Walking hamstring stretch** - Perform the dynamic stretch while walking for 10 yards or meters. Bend at the waist, holding your forward leg straight and reach your hands toward the ground by your forward foot with each step. Keep the non-stretching knee bent slightly for stability as you stretch.

2. **Walking groiner stretch** - Perform this dynamic stretch while striding forward for 10 yards or meters. For each lunging stride, take a big step as if you're performing a lunge and drop your back knee toward the ground. As you settle into the stretch, keep your head up as you bring your chest toward your extended knee. Place both hands on the ground so you don't lose balance as you stretch. Lean forward as needed to bring the stretch deeper into your hamstrings and glutes.

3. **Walking quad stretch** - Perform the stretch while walking forward for 10 meters or yards. While standing, take one foot and pull it upward toward your buttocks. Alternating legs, drop your foot, take one step forward, and then repeat the quad stretch.

4. **Low hurdle running drill** - Perform the exercise for 25 meters or yards. Run forward and imagine you're running over a low, 4 to 6-inch (10 to 15 centimeter) high hurdle with each step.

5. **High hurdle running drill** - Perform the warmup exercise for 25 meters or yards. Run forward and visualize striding over a 12-inch (1/3 meter) high hurdle with each step.

6. **Leg swings** - Perform 10 swings per leg, swinging your legs front to back and side to side. When swinging your legs,

stand upright, keep your leg straight, and hold onto something stable. Swing each leg 10 times backward and forward and then 10 times side to side while maintaining good form. Switch legs when complete.

The Workout:

1. **Uphill sprint** - Run uphill for 10 seconds, roughly 25 to 50 meters or yards, this will help reduce lactic acid buildup in your legs. Use 80 to 100 percent of your maximum effort when sprinting.
2. **Repeat** - Perform the hill sprint 6 times using good form while fully engaging your muscles, especially your calves.

Ramping Intensity Sprint Program:

Implementing many variations for your hill workouts will build your calves. Here's a graduated routine that builds in intensity going farther and higher over time, while reducing set volume for longer distances:

1. 5 sprints x 10 meters or yards, rest for 15 seconds between sprints.
2. 4 sprints x 20 meters or yards, rest for 30 seconds between sprints.

3. 3 sprints x 30 meters or yards, rest for 60 seconds between sprints.
4. 2 sprints x 40 meters or yards, rest for 90 seconds between sprints.
5. 1 sprint x 50 plus meters or yards. Go farther if the hill is long enough and you're ready to challenge yourself.

Remember, the emphasis when sprinting is on exercise quality despite the high exertion. To give adequate recovery time, the rest periods between sets increases with each new distance. The better your form and the more engaged you are in your movements, the better your results… be intense but maintain good form!

Reduce your volume and intensity if you are inexperienced with sprinting. As you get fitter, increase the distances, variation, and intensity—or decrease the rest intervals—to help prevent plateauing. For example, run longer, harder, use a steeper hill, or add weight to continue overloading your muscles. In addition to more developed calves, be prepared for some serious back, leg, and core development as well as a leaner overall physique.

The Never-Ending Sets Workout:

This hill program relies on increasing the number, intensity, and length of sprints as your strength and endurance increases.

As you adjust to this method of high-volume sprint training, the running intervals become longer, increasing in duration to 10 to 12 seconds per sprint. When beginning, look for a hill about 40 meters or yards long. Find a bigger hill as needed.

Warmup:

To warm up for your sprints, do cardio, light jogging, and dynamic stretches for roughly 10 to 15 minutes. Short jogs, leg swings, jumping jacks, skips, and squats are good examples of exercises to help you get ready.

The workout:

1. When you feel ready, perform five uphill sprints at roughly 70 to 80 percent of maximal effort over roughly 40 meters or yards.
2. Shake out your legs to remain loose and let yourself recover as you walk down the hill after each sprint.
3. Finish your workout with a 10-to-15 minute cool down using exercises and stretches similar to those used for the warmup.
4. As you train and improve, gradually increase your sprints' length, intensity, and number by one or two sprints per week until you've progressed to 20 at maximal effort over a longer distance. Each sprint should take about 10 seconds to complete.

The Mountain:

This program is as simple as it is grueling. Find a hill, the bigger and steeper the better, but one that you can run up. Bring something heavy, such as a weight vest, a sandbag, a loaded backpack, a bag of dog food, last year's tax forms, or whatever works. Warm up thoroughly. Once you're ready, holding your weight securely, run up the hill as fast as you can. When you can't run, walk. When you can't walk, scramble and crawl.

If you don't have a long, steep hill nearby, use a treadmill set on maximum gradient.

If you don't have a treadmill, use stairs. You will need enough flights to push yourself to your limits.

The goal of the mountain is to reach absolute failure in a single set. Use good form and push through with your calves with each step—as long as you're able—while your muscles and form slowly deteriorate.

The Mountain is not a workout to be undertaken lightly. It is intended to push and test your limits... two key factors in both physical and mental growth.

Hill Sprint Tips & Tricks:

1. If your hill is close to your home, consider walking, jogging, or bicycling to the hill as a warm-up. Then walk, jog, or cycle back home as a cool-down.
2. If you find your sprinting area has poor traction, consider a pair of track shoes or cleats to improve your grip.
   Alternatively, if your hill is part of a trail, you may want to

purchase trail running shoes to maintain good footing and provide ankle support.

3. Use whatever hill(s) you have nearby to set your target sprint distances. If you have two or more hills close, create separate workouts for each hill. Alternatively, adjust the length of your sprint workouts each week based on the hills available—long and short hill-sprinting sessions.

4. Time your sprints with a stopwatch. To help prevent injury, when your times decrease by 10 percent or more, stop your session for the day.

5. Because of their intensity, allow yourself adequate time to recover between hill workouts.

6. As your strength and stamina increase, add more sprints per session.

7. Try other sprint programs to add variety, intensity, and prevent plateauing.

8. To make your sessions more intense, add weight. Weight vests are a nice option, particularly those that offer adjustable weight ranges. Start low and work up to higher weights.

9. Hills also offer great opportunities for other exercises, so consider adding them to your routine since you've already come this far. Options include hill jumps—jumping up the hill for quads and glutes—decline crunches, bear crawls up and down the hill, and incline/decline push-ups. Now that you've found your hill, make the most of it!

10. Use variations in how you sprint. Run pushing up from the ground using a full range of motion in your feet to emphasize calf engagement. As an alternative, stay on your toes as you run. Mix techniques to keep your muscles firing and prevent your calves from adapting.

11. If you don't have access to hills, stairs, a treadmill, or if you just want some variety in your program, consider doing any of these hill sprint workouts on flat ground.

Hill sprinting is a powerful tool to bring to your calf-training arsenal. Not only will you get outside for a change of scenery and pace, but also, your calves will never know what hit them.

SIFF LUNGES AND SIFF SQUATS FOR DIAMOND CALVES

If you're frustrated about not getting your desired results in your calves even though you work your legs diligently, have I got an exercise variation for you!

Siff lunges and Siff squats!

Here's a program that will put your calves under pressure, polish them, and eventually turn them into diamonds:

Siff lunges - Siff lunges are a unique lunge variation where you always stay on the tips of your toes. To perform a Siff lunge, elevate off your heels and remain on your toes throughout the exercise. Siff lunges can also be performed plyometrically as well for an intensified variation—jumping up and down through your lunges while remaining on your toes throughout the movement. For your Siff lunge routine, perform:

1. **Sets**: 3-4.

2. **Reps**: 8-10 per side.
3. **Rest**: 90 seconds between sets.

Standing calf raises - Perform your standing calf raises on a calf-raise machine, using a squat bar, on a seated leg press machine, or with dumbbells... whatever makes you work. For your standing calf raises, perform:

1. 2 sets of 6 to 8 reps with your feet in the neutral, forward-facing position.
2. 2 sets of 6 to 8 reps with your feet and toes turned outward.
3. 2 sets of 6 to 8 reps with your feet and toes turned inward.

Be sure to start each repetition from a pause in the stretched position. For added burn, pause at the peak contraction as well.

Seated calf raises - Perform your seated calf raises on a seated calf raise machine. If you don't have access to a seated calf machine, use a chair, elevating your heels off the ground using a plate, bar, or other flat object and rest the weights on your knees to lift. Alternatively, squat down with your knees completely bent and your buttocks resting on your heels, and perform calf raises from the seated squat position. For your seated calf raises, perform:

1. **Sets**: 3.
2. **Reps**: Perform 30 total repetitions. Do 10 reps with your feet

and toes turned inward, 10 reps with your feet and toes in a neutral, forward-facing position, and 10 reps with your feet and toes turned outward.

Notes:

1. Each set of seated calf raises has a total of 30 repetitions.
2. For the seated and standing calf raises, start each rep from a stretched position at the bottom of the lift and hold the peak top contraction for at least two seconds.

Perform this calf-burning routine two to three times per week.

If your calves have lost their luster, this routine will put some shine on those gems.

Bonus Siff Exercise:

For an added bonus, throw in Siff squats on your leg day(s) to get your calves screaming.

How to Siff Squat:

• • •

Start your leg workouts with Siff squats. Siff squats are performed exactly like regular squats with two exceptions: you stay on the balls of your feet while squatting and you use a slightly lighter weight than in a normal squat.

To do your Siff squats, use 75 to 85 percent of the weight you would typically use for a standard squat. Start your set as you would for a normal squat with the bar resting on your shoulders. After getting into the start position, raise your heels off the ground so that you're standing on the balls of your feet. Use a block or bar if needed as a guide to help keep your heels off the ground or for stability. Perform a squat, keeping your heels elevated for the entire movement.

Perform 2 to 3 sets of 8 to 10 reps each. Rest for two minutes between sets. Stay on your toes as much as possible to engage your calves and stability muscles.

Why the Siff Squat Works:

The classic squat is one of the best overall total body-building exercises because it engages numerous muscle groups for maximum stimulus and hormone release. In addition to all the benefits of traditional squats, Siff squats force your calves to support a heavier load than normal, providing a powerful stimulus for growth. Siff squats also add additional stress and growth opportunities for your quads because raising your heels forces your center of gravity and weight slightly forward during exertion.

The dynamic Siff squat can help strengthen your weak points and push your body to its limits.

JUMP FOR JOY FOR YOUR CALVES

Jumping explosively can be great for your calves and body in general. Plyometrics—jumping exercises—are an excellent tool to increase strength, explosive power, and muscle mass. Here are a few calf-focused plyometric exercises to push your calves in new directions and help them grow.

These exercises can be worked into your calf routine, incorporated into your leg days, or used together to build a routine of their own. Alternatively, add them with other plyometric exercises to boost your overall leg strength and power.

Be careful when performing jumping exercises as they put quite a lot of pressure and stress on your joints and body. As with sprints, warm up thoroughly before beginning plyometric training. Listen to your body and take precautions to reduce injury risk. Taking precautions such as jumping on a mat or grass and using good form can all reduce impact pressures.

. . .

Ankle Jumps:

Ankle jumps are a classic calf workout that is both explosive and athletic. When doing ankle jumps, take inspiration from sprinters, dancers, and gymnasts. Ankle jumps mimic these athletes' explosive activity, taking your calves to new heights.

Here's how:

1. Stand with your feet together with your arms relaxed and your hands resting loosely by your sides.
2. Keeping your legs as straight as possible, jump up and down from a single spot by pushing explosively off your toes. Jump as high as possible with maximum effort and exertion. Do not let your heels touch down onto the ground between jumps.
3. Continue jumping until your calves burn and your form starts to become compromised.
4. Rest and repeat until failure.

Tips and Variations:

1. Jump from side to side to work the lateral sides of your calves.
2. To increase the intensity of the workout, incorporate any of

the methods listed. Increasing the number of reps or sets, try hopping on one leg, wearing a weighted vest, jumping higher, or holding dumbbells while carrying out your jumps.

3. Remember, ankle jumps are not a squat jump or normal leap. Avoid bending at the knees as much as possible when performing your ankle jumps to keep the focus of your exertion in your calf muscles as much as possible.

Jumping Rope:

If you want to take your calves to new heights, jump into plyometrics for a world of exercises to push yourself to new limits. Jumping rope is a plyometric classic where you can isolate your calves to your heart's content. Although typically associated with adding definition to your calves and legs in general, jumping rope can also build your calves depending on your program and goals. When jumping, use a full range of motion and focus primarily on your calves to get better muscle engagement and improved results.

Basic Jump Rope Routine:

To start your jump rope workouts, consider alternating between 30 seconds of work with 30 seconds of rest. Taken together, each exercise and rest cycle makes one round. Do 10 to 20 rounds in total, choosing from the jump rope variations outlined below.

As you progress, perform each exercise for a minute or more with shorter rests in between. Build up your exertion phases as your skill, endurance, and strength grow. Harder exercises like double-unders may be more difficult to sustain for the designated time. Just do your best and keep working.

Jump Rope Variations:

1. **Basic Jump** - The classic jump rope option. Simply jump up and down in place as you swing the rope around and under your feet. The basic jump is easy to perform and doing it for longer intervals will get a good calf burn. Adjust the height and speed of your jumps to increase intensity.
2. **Front-to-Back** - Jump forward and backward as you jump over the rope. With this jump, your body has to dynamically stabilize as you're moving your feet forwards and backwards. This movement gives your calves an extra challenge, targeting more muscle fibers.
3. **Side-to-Side** - Jump from side to side laterally while jumping over the rope. Side jumps improve your lateral speed and explosiveness. These explosive movements can improve muscle definition and density.
4. **Alternating Foot Steps** - Alternate between landing on each foot as you jump from one leg to the other while jumping over the rope. This variation is performed as if you are running in place. The quick tempo helps improve your calves' reaction time.
5. **High Knee Step** - Perform alternating jumps over the rope as you would with alternating foot step jumps, except with

this variation, raise your feet and knees higher, aiming for knees bent with thighs parallel to the ground. This is a higher impact exercise, so it improves calf strength.

6. **Single-Leg Jumps** - Jump up and down on one leg without alternating between feet. Single-leg jumps are great for explosiveness and strength because you're putting all of your bodyweight and impact energy on one leg, isolating each calf. All the energy involved in jumping on one leg will also work your feet and ankles.

7. **Double-Unders** - Jump into the air high enough to swing the jump rope beneath your feet twice before landing. The higher jumps from double-unders will improve power and explosiveness.

8. **Mummy Kicks** - Alternate kicking your feet out forward as you jump and stay on the balls of your feet and toes the whole time. With mummy kicks, your feet kick outward with legs mostly straight and then return to their starting position below the body in preparation to jump outward again. This exercise is calf muscle intensive. Focus on contracting your calves every time your feet hit the ground.

As with any jumping exercise, consider adding weight, such as with a weighted vest or increasing your jumping height to increase intensity. If needed, try jumping on a mat or other soft surface to reduce the stress of impact on your joints.

Jump Rope Circuit Routine:

. . .

There's a wealth of options to choose from to create a calf-burning jump rope workout. Here's a great circuit incorporating the jump rope variations.

Do the following exercises in a complete circuit 2 or 3 times. Rest for 10 seconds in between each jump rope exercise in the circuit before moving on to the next movement.

1. 30-second basic jump – a standard two-footed jump.
2. 30-second alternating footsteps – jump as though you're running in place.
3. 60-second single-leg jumps – 30-second jump on one leg before switching to the other leg for a further 30 seconds.
4. 30-second mummy kicks – kicking feet forward as you jump.
5. 30-second double-unders – rotate the rope twice with each jump.
6. 30-second single leg double-unders – 30 seconds with each leg. If you can't do single leg double-unders, repeat the double leg double-unders or do more single leg jumps.

Add variations to keep challenging yourself and to increase the intensity. Again, adding a weight vest and higher jumps will also push your calves harder.

Explosive, Nonjumping Calf Exercise Routine:

• • •

You don't have to jump off the ground to mimic the explosive exertions of leaping into the air. This routine mimics the forceful movements and dynamic pressures associated with leaping and sprinting to blast your calves into the strata.

Be sure to keep your knees straight but not locked out during each of these exercises.

Single-Leg Explosive Calf Raises:

1. Stand on a block, stair, or platform with the heel of one foot hanging over the edge.
2. Slowly lower your heel while keeping your knee straight.
3. Explosively extend your ankle upward as far as your range of motion allows, pushing upward through the ball of your foot and onto your toes as you lift.
4. Be sure to pause at the bottom of the exercise to reduce Achilles tendon involvement and encourage full muscle engagement.
5. Perform 3 sets for each leg with 6 to 8 explosive reps per set.

Single-Leg Hurdle Jumps:

1. Place 6 to 8 agility or speed-training hurdles in a straight line along the ground. Set each hurdle roughly 2 feet (2/3 of a meter) apart. If you don't have hurdles, visualize jumping over a low object—about one to three inches / two to eight

centimeters above the ground—as you bounce forward. Alternatively, place other small objects on the ground to jump over.
2. On one leg, jump over the hurdles one at a time without pausing between jumps, traveling over the hurdles as quickly as possible.
3. Perform 2 to 3 sets with 6 to 8 repetitions for each leg. Do all the jumps in a set with the same leg before switching to the other leg.

Single-Leg Box Jumps:

1. Stand on one leg with a 4 to 6-inch (10 to 15 centimeter) box, block, or step in front of you.
2. Jump up onto the box, powerfully forcing your foot downward to generate power and upward momentum.
3. Jump down and quickly explode upward again to repeat.
4. Perform 3 sets with 6 to 8 repetitions for each leg.

For each of these exercises, consider adding height or weight for additional intensity.

These are but a few of the many jumping exercises that will blast your calves. For more ideas, take inspiration from your childhood when you jumped and skipped for fun. Also, look to track athletes' plyometric training, particularly those of sprinters, long-jumpers, and high-jumpers for additional ideas. Basketball drills, particularly those with a plyometric emphasis, are another great source of ideas for plyometric training.

Now go out and get jumping for those calf gains!

BLOOD FLOW RESTRICTION TO RELEASE CALF GROWTH

This book is full of exercises and ideas to help you get a skin-splitting amount of blood flowing to your calves. Choices to torture your legs and get those calves to grow include high volume training, explosive training, heavy training, drop sets, reverse drop sets, supersets, partial sets, plyometrics, and numerous others.

But one of the most effective ways to influence your muscles' pump is through blood flow restriction (BFR) or occlusion training.

Knee wraps offer a simple, easily accessible means to use BFR training on the calves. Simply apply the wraps just below the knee, right above where the gastrocnemius muscle meets the knee joint. Tighten the wraps about 30 to 40 percent looser than you would for a set of squats. Experiment with the tension until the tightness feels most comfortable to you, especially if you have never used wraps before.

Wrapping makes each set more challenging. If you wrap your calves too tightly, you'll never complete a full set—you have been warned!

Use any exercise or machine to train with your legs wrapped, including seated calf raises, donkey calf raises, horizontal calf extensions, or standing calf raises.

If you're truly working, be prepared to test your physical and mental limits when you exercise your calves using BFR.

When working your calves with BFR, aim for three sets of 10 to 15 repetitions with 30-second rest breaks in between each set. The intensity of the burn you'll get with BFR calf training will challenge your resolve. To help with recovery and calf development, be sure to stretch in between sets and after—massage, heat, cold packs, and electrical muscle stimulation are other valuable recovery options.

Here's a basic overview of how BFR training works:

1. Do 10 to 15 full range reps.
2. Stand and rest/stretch for 30 seconds.
3. Perform another set of 10 to 15 reps.
4. Rest/stretch another 30 seconds.
5. Finish with a final set of 10 to 15 reps.
6. Then remove the wraps.

Work up to three rounds of these calf killers.

When undertaking BFR training, don't forget the second key to calf hypertrophy—stretching. A good 30-second stretch of each calf at the end of each set of BFR is both painful and vital.

Since you're performing standard calf raises with your legs wrapped, consider any variation presented in this book to increase the intensity of your exercise or shift the emphasis as you train with BFR —rep timing and cadence, contractions, pauses, weight amount, number of reps, rep explosivity or wrap tightness. If lifting heavier weights, consider dropping the number of reps as well.

Your calves will thank me when you're done… once the pain subsides.

MORE CALF ROUTINES AND TECHNIQUES

I hope *Killer Calves* has your brain bursting with ideas of ways to boost and enhance your calf development. I also hope this book has inspired you to become just as stubborn as your calves and willing to do everything you possibly can to get them to grow without giving up.

Additionally, I hope that the programs and variations in *Killer Calves* have given you enough information to begin exploring new calf-blasting routines of your own.

However, in case you need more, here are a few bonus calf-destroying programs to keep you pushing, and calf raising to your ultimate goals—killer calves.

The Two-Minute Calf Raise

· · ·

This standing calf-raise routine aims to maximize your benefits from using the standing calf-raise machine, helping you overcome bad habits or poor form you may have developed in the past.

This routine requires you to leave your ego at the door. As you get stronger, you'll eventually be able to add more weight and find other ways to intensify the routine.

Here's how:

1. Choose a weight 50 to 75% lighter than you would generally use for a set of 10 to 15 reps.
2. Do your first rep with a nice hard contraction at the highest point of your lift, and then lower your heels until you're in a complete stretch at the bottom of the lift. <u>Important</u>: You are constantly controlling the weight on the way down and not dropping it. Actively resist the weight pushing down into the calves as you lower, feeling the weight in your calves as you move. Hold the stretched bottom position for at least 10 seconds. Use a clock if you have to but don't cut your time short!
3. Now do another long, controlled rep. That means raise up, squeeze tightly, control the weight down to full extension, and hold at the bottom for another full 10-second stretch.
4. Perform 12 to 15 of these slow, controlled repetitions. If you performed the reps properly, your calves will have been under two minutes or more of unrelenting tension.
5. Perform 3 total sets of slow, extended calf raises.
6. Wonder when you'll be able to walk again. Just kidding… walking and stretching will help relieve the soreness and

stiffness. And the pain will remind you why you're putting yourself through this torture.

7. For variations, consider holding the contractions at the top of your raise longer, adding additional weight, or increasing the number of reps performed.

Sprinting Intervals

As an alternative to hill sprints, consider doing sprinting intervals on flat ground.

Why, you might ask?

The powerful legs of sprinters can rival those of some bodybuilders. Sprinting is an anaerobic exercise, meaning sprints do not rely on oxygen consumption during exertion and mainly utilize fast-twitch muscle fibers. Sprinting creates an ideal framework for calf growth since sprinting requires rapid deceleration which results in powerful eccentric muscle contractions. It also harnesses significant power with each explosive movement and utilizes rapid acceleration, creating forceful concentric contractions as your legs propel your body. In addition to calf growth, sprinting will also give you further muscular development in your quads, hamstrings, glutes, and core, as well as improving your cardiovascular resilience.

How to Sprint:

· · ·

The biomechanics of sprinting are a bit different than regular running or jogging. With traditional jogging, you are striking the ground heel to toe with each stride. In contrast, sprinting will have you striking the ground with your toes first. This toe-first strike is where the eccentric contraction of the calf muscles comes in. Depending on your speed and form, you may or may not even touch your heels to the ground during sprints.

When sprinting, focus on landing on your toes instead of your heels. Perform a series of intervals with a moderate to high work-to-rest ratio—short exertions and longer rests. For example, you might sprint for 10 to 20 seconds at maximum speed and rest for 2 to 3 minutes between each sprint.

For variations, perform any of the hill sprint routines—mentioned previously—on flat ground, add weight, increase sprint distance, incorporate plyometrics, or reduce the rest time between sets.

Seated Calf Scorchers

If you like to work your calves at the end of your workout but your legs are so burned out that you can barely stand, then this timed seated calf raise workout is for you.

Here's how:

1. On the seated calf machine, perform as many repetitions as you can in a full minute. You are not counting reps. You are pushing yourself hard for a full minute.

2. Use good form and a controlled eccentric—negative downward movement.
3. Do not stop exercising for the entire minute.
4. Do at least 2 sets, focusing on getting the maximum amount of work in each minute.
5. Get a fire extinguisher ready to put out your calves. Or stretch. I recommend stretching.
6. Add more weight, change the angles of your feet, or increase the exercise duration, which will increase the number of reps performed, to intensify the set.

2-day Trauma

If you want your calves to grow, to be strong, and give your body foundational stability, then this 2-day program is just what you need.

You'll perform this calf routine twice a week, and also take a 48-hour break between the High and Low Volume sections. Session 1 focuses on low weight with high volume. Session 2 focuses on heavy weight with low volume. Both routines will light your calves on fire. And, combined, they will help your calves grow.

Here's how:

Day 1 - High-Volume

The high-volume day consists of two separate supersets.

Perform the seated calf raises and donkey calf raises detailed below in succession with a 10-second rest between each exercise to make the first high-volume superset. Rest for 2 minutes between supersets. Repeat the seated calf raises and donkey calf raises in sequence for a total of 3 supersets using the appropriate number of reps for that set.

Move to the standing calf raise for 10 sets using a 10-second break between sets as explained below.

Seated Calf Raises - Perform 3 sets x 10-5-5 reps, respectively. This means you'll do 10 reps in the first set, then 5 reps in both the second and third sets. Use a 1-0-1 rhythm for your lifts. That means you will take 1 second to lower the weight down. You will not pause at the bottom of the lift. And you will take 1 second to raise the weight back up.

Donkey Calf Raises - Do 3 sets x 30-50 reps in each set. Perform each lift with a 1-0-1 rhythm, as explained above.

Standing Calf Raises - Perform 10 sets x 10-30 reps each set. Use a 1-1-1 tempo for each lift. This means you will take 1 second to lower the weight. You will pause for 1 second at the bottom of the lift. Then you'll take 1 second to lift the weight back up. Rest 10 seconds between sets.

Day 2 - Low-Volume

Perform the Day-2 low-volume routine 48 hours after the Day-1 high-volume routine.

Triple Drop Set Standing Calf Raises - Do 3 sets x 10-10-10 reps, respectively. You will perform 3 drop sets of 10 reps per drop set, for 30 total reps in each complete set. Each drop set will use a successively lower weight. Each rep is done at a 1-2-1 rhythm. Rest 90 seconds between sets.

Be sure to take the full 2-second pause at the bottom of the lift.

• • •

Given the intensity of these routines, be sure to stretch thoroughly.

Anti-Arnold Donkey Calf Raises

First of all, I am not Anti-Arnold. I love Arnold and especially his pioneering calf training. But Arnold is also known for loading several sweaty men onto his back for his donkey calf raises. I'm offering cleaner, less sweaty alternatives.

The magic of the donkey calf raise is that your calf muscles, particularly your gastrocnemius muscles, are forced into an ideal, fully stretched position at the bottom of the exercise. This fully stretched position makes you engage as many muscle fibers as possible when lifting.

Here are a few options for performing donkey calf raises:

1. If you don't have access to a donkey calf raise machine at your gym, strap on a loaded dipping belt and stand on a stable, elevated block with your toes on the edge of the block. Alternatively, use a Smith machine squat rack.
2. If using a dipping belt, bend at the waist, letting the weight hang between your legs. If using a Smith machine or donkey calf raise machine, bend at the waist, engage the weight on the bar, and let the weight rest—wherever it's comfortable—on your lower back, so that the weight drives directly down your legs.
3. Perform the donkey calf raises with your legs straight and

the weight driving directly down through your legs and into your heels.

4. Make sure you are maximizing your range of movement. This means your feet will be traveling through a full range of motion with each repetition.

5. Your donkey calf raises can be performed in a bilateral or unilateral position with one or two legs. If using one leg, find something suitable to hold or rest on to maintain balance.

6. Use any rep ranges, weight setups, numbers of sets, contraction timing, or exercise variations required to fully fatigue your calves. See the *Variations* chapter for ideas.

For those working out at home, also think about donkey calf raises without summoning family members to sit on your back—if they're willing to help, then you're already good to go—all you need is a dog leash and dumbbells or weight plates.

Loop the leash around the dumbbell(s) or through the hole in the weight plate(s). Fasten the leash clamp around the leash's handle to make a loop. Step through the resulting loop, adjust the leash to rest around your hips, bend over, and let the weight hang between your legs. Now begin lifting!

Fascial Release and Other Recovery Techniques

• • •

If you're doing everything right and still not seeing the calf development you're after, you may want to try Active Release Therapy (ART) and similar massage programs.

Weight training and other demanding physical activities can lead to soft tissue damage over time. Tightness of the fascia—the supportive connective tissues surrounding your muscles, organs, bones, and blood vessels and which help hold them in place—may restrict muscle growth. Proper treatment of these damaged tissues with ART may help release these constraining tissues, allowing muscle growth to take place.

Here's one way to perform active release therapy for your calves on your own:

1. Sit on the floor or ground with one leg bent and the other straight.
2. On the elevated, bent leg, hold your calf with both hands. Place your thumbs on your shin with your fingers wrapped around your lower calf. While applying pressure with your hands, straighten your leg and flex your toes as your elevated leg comes to rest beside your supporting leg.
3. Return the formerly elevated leg to the starting position. Bend your leg and move your fingers up it to the middle of your calf. As before, apply pressure, and extend your leg with your toes pointed as you return it to the floor.
4. Repeat the same dynamic massage on the upper part of your calf.
5. Repeat the progressive massage on the inside and the outside of the muscle, starting from the bottom and working your way up, massaging the bottom, middle, and top portions of your calf as you extend your leg and point your toes.

6. Repeat the same procedure for the other leg.

Don't be limited to ART to help your body grow, release tension, and recover. Other techniques and approaches can provide positive recovery and preventative benefits such as:

1. Stretching, both dynamic and static.
2. Pressure, trigger point, and percussive self-massage.
3. Assisted massage—deep tissue, sports massage, shiatsu massage, lymphatic massage or reflexology.
4. Ice bath, cold water immersion or cold shower therapy.
5. Various relaxation, meditation, and visualization techniques.

HIIT Those Calves

High intensity training is generally considered to be training involving periods of exercise at or near maximal exertion followed by short periods of rest. These rest periods generally do not provide enough time for full recovery from the intense exertion.

Tabata training, for example, is one type of HIIT training method where you go through one or more exercises over a 4-minute period. Tabatas involve 8 x 20-second exertion phases and 8 x 10-second rest phases. So, over 4 minutes, you exert yourself at or near maximum effort for 20 seconds and then take a 10-second break 8 times in the 4-minute Tabata set.

Tabatas and HIIT can make great calf-building challenges. They allow you to put your calves through short, intense bursts of exertion. You could, for example, mix up as many calf exercises as you can think of in a single HIIT session or just focus on one.

One of my favorite HIIT sessions involves drop-set Tabatas with standing calf raises. If you don't have access to a calf-raise machine, use a weight vest or dumbbells as an alternative. After warming up for 20 seconds, perform normal single or double-legged calf raises with the maximum weight you can handle for 8 to 12 reps. When you can no longer lift that weight with good form, drop to a lower weight —during the rest cycles—and keep pushing in the active phases.

If your calves are not on fire after 8 successive sets with minimal rest between, you're not trying hard enough, not using enough weight, or using bad form.

HIIT training pushes you to your limits in short, intense time periods. As such, you may need significant recovery time after HIIT sessions. But your calves won't know what hit them.

The Challenge

This is a simple exercise intended to push your limits, much like the Mountain. This routine is also great incorporated into other programs or as a separate workout.

The Challenge is simple: perform as many single-leg calf raises as you can with each leg. Use good form controlling the motion—without bouncing—making sure to pause at the bottom and top of each rep.

Use a step, a curb, a suitable rock, or anything else that will let you move through a complete motion. When you're unable to perform any more complete repetitions, continue with partial reps, performing partial contractions as high as you're able to press upward.

Finished with one leg? Then switch to the other. Set a goal and go for it!

Once you've hit that goal, go for more!

As usual, consider intensifying the routine and throwing off your body's adaptations by increasing reps, slowing down reps, holding your stretch and contractions for longer at the bottom and top of your reps, adding weight, and any other variation that pushes you that bit further. As an alternative, perform the Challenge with both legs simultaneously instead of one leg at a time.

Climbing the Mountain

What happens when you cross The Challenge with The Mountain?

You climb the mountain!

Climbing the Mountain is another basic calf exercise challenge. Perform it doing either single or double-leg calf raises. Here's how Climbing the Mountain works. Find a set of stairs. If you don't have stairs, a single step—or sturdy object—will do, but you may lose some sense of accomplishment as you climb without visible upward movement and progress. Choose a number of reps to perform on each set, then climb away!

You'll do that number of repetitions on each step for each leg, individually or both at the same time. Once you've performed those repetitions, you go up to the next step.

Keep climbing, or repeating if you don't have access to stairs, until you have to stop and cannot climb any farther.

Choose whatever calf-raise variation(s) you want or change them as you climb—

extended peak contractions, extended calf stretches, explosive lifts, partial rep pauses, adding weight, extending the concentric and/or eccentric movement. Do whatever you can to challenge yourself and shock your muscles into growth as you move. Once you've reached your limits, remember how far you climbed and then try to surpass those limits the next time you climb the mountain!

As with the other approaches presented in *Killer Calves*, the important thing with these routines is to explore, experiment, and ultimately find what works for you. Once you've found what works, keep pushing to learn and do more.

Good luck and may the gains be with you!

WHAT'S NEXT?

The honest answer to that question is the next steps in your calf training and development are up to you. Just as you determine how hard you work and how much success you have, you will determine how much your calves grow and how well they are maintained.

Personally, I exercise my calves two to three times a day, every day. This is the level of commitment required for me to see results. Since I started working with this level of dedication, my calves—and I'm a hard gainer—have grown.

They are now larger than my biceps.

However, I know that if I stop exercising hard, varying my routines, and challenging myself, I will not see additional growth. I also know that if I do not work to maintain what I have gained, this progress will gradually disappear. With any luck, your road is much easier than mine.

But, whatever your journey, *Killer Calves* will get you there.

So, the choice is yours. *Killer Calves* offers you the tools needed to help you achieve the calves of your dreams, and hopefully the ideas presented here have inspired you to push and strive for your goals.

Remember, your calves, like your life, are what you make of them.

I want you to keep pushing, to never stop exploring, and to continually develop.

Then, your calves won't be the only thing that are killer.

—Rhys Larson

HELP SPREAD THE WORD!

Thank you for taking the time to pick up and read my calf development guide. I hope you found *Killer Calves* worthwhile and that you will crush your calf goals as a result.

If you appreciated this book, please help spread the word and consider leaving a review.

Everyone needs killer calves.

Together, with your help, we can make that possible.

Many thanks—and many gains!

—Rhys Larson

CITATIONS

Here are the sources for the quotes used in *Killer Calves*:

1. "The Complete Arnold: Calves." *Muscle & Fitness*, 9 June 2017, www.muscleandfitness.com/flexonline/training/complete-arnold-calves/.
2. "Lou Ferrigno's Mass Class." *Muscle & Fitness*, 29 Dec. 2015, www.muscleandfitness.com/flexonline/training/lou-ferrignos-mass-class/.
3. Old School Labs. *Secret to Historic Calves | Q&A with Golden Era Legend Tom Platz.* www.youtube.com/watch?v=yiJqIRoXVfk.
4. Ladon, Jacob. "This Mass Monster Has Some of the Craziest Monster Calves in Bodybuilding History." *Generation Iron Fitness & Bodybuilding Network*, 12 July 2019,

generationiron.com/this-mass-monster-has-some-of-the-craziest-monster-calves-in-bodybuilding-history/.

5. "Want Calves Like Flex Lewis?" *Muscle & Fitness*, 19 July 2012, www.muscleandfitness.com/flexonline/training/want-calves-flex-lewis/.

SYNOPSIS

Not everyone is born with the calves of their dreams. Whether you want calves that are well-formed, defined, supple, huge, or ripped, *Killer Calves* can help make your dreams a reality.

For those who want to banish their chicken legs to the distant past, *Killer Calves* will help turn shrimpy calves into raging bulls.

If you want to be fit, bring variety to your exercise routines, add some lower leg development, or maintain what you have already worked so hard to attain, *Killer Calves* is for you too.

Killer Calves offers a wide range of tools, exercises, insights, and ideas to help shape your legs, particularly your calves.

So, if you're a hard gainer who has tried everything—or think you have—to build your calves, *Killer Calves* will give you numerous new ways to push your limits and help your muscles grow. If you're looking to sculpt and tone your lower legs, *Killer Calves* will provide you with a host of options to achieve the look you're after. Or, if you're already jacked and looking to add a bit of variety and new options to your leg routine, *Killer Calves* will give you novel ideas and programs to torture yourself at home and the gym.

Whether you're a fitness beginner looking for help, a seasoned bodybuilder or fitness professional looking for that little edge, someone who wants to get in shape, or an exercise enthusiast looking for a new approach, *Killer Calves* will help you improve your legs.

Everyone deserves a great pair of legs.

Everyone deserves a pair of killer calves!

www.ingramcontent.com/pod-product-compliance
Lightning Source LLC
Chambersburg PA
CBHW031310250726
48656CB00005B/1723